HARDCORE
KETTLEBELL
TRAINING
FOR
MEN

Published by Price World Publishing
3971 Hoover Rd. Suite 77
Columbus, OH 43123-2839
www.PriceWorldPublishing.com

Cover Design by Russell Marleau
Layout Design by Merwin Loquias
Editing by Rob Price
Printing by United Graphics

ISBN: 978-1-932549-867
eBook ISBN: 9781619844179
Library of Congress Control Number: 2014952172

Printed in the United States of America
10 9 8 7 6 5 4 3 2 1

For information about discounts for bulk purchases, please contact info@priceworldpublishing.com.

HARDCORE KETTLEBELL TRAINING FOR MEN

JIM McHALE

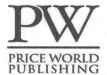

PW
PRICE WORLD
PUBLISHING

Dedication

This book is dedicated to all those who strive to constantly improve themselves. Stay Hungry!

"The resistance that you fight physically in the gym and the resistance that you fight in life can only build a strong character."

— Arnold Schwarzenegger

ACKNOWLEDGEMENTS

I was able to write this book because of so many people.

First, a huge thank you to my parents for instilling in me the values that will always guide me.

Thank you also to:

My sister, Victoria, and her family for their love and support.

My friend, Dan, for his consistent advice and guidance.

My friend, Terry, for sharing his expert training and nutrition knowledge.

CONTENTS

INTRODUCTION

A SHORT INTRODUCTION TO KETTLEBELLS

The fundamental goal of this book is to act as an **easy-to-use guide to training with kettlebells**. Whether you have used kettlebells before or you are just starting out, the exercises and workouts included in these pages will show you how to get the absolute most out of your training.

Above all this book is intended to help you enjoy training with kettlebells while delivering the results that you desire. Whether you want to get supremely fit and explosive, build muscle, or burn fat, proper use of the kettlebell can help.

So what exactly is a kettlebell? It is a simple yet extremely effective piece of gym equipment; a cast-iron weight with a handle. That's it!

Kettlebells were invented in Russia several centuries ago and were used extensively by the Soviet army in physical-training programs in the 20th Century. More recently they have seen a surge in popularity with personal trainers and athletes of all types. Walk into almost any gym these days and you will see a variety of kettlebells.

Most kettlebell weight loads increase in 4kg increments, though you can find them in pretty much any size if you look hard enough. They typically range from 2kg to over 32kg each. It is extremely important that you choose weight loads that are good for you and are prepared to vary the weights for different exercises and circuits listed in this book.

Kettlebells can be purchased in most physical sporting goods stores and online. Prices can vary quite a lot depending on the quality of manufacture and materials. Compared to expensive gym memberships, kettlebells offer excellent value. They are great to keep at home and take up very little space, especially compared to other home gym equipment such as exercise bikes, treadmills, and even barbells.

HOW THIS BOOK WILL HELP DELIVER THE RESULTS YOU WANT

The main use for kettlebells is to perform **dynamic exercises**, which combine cardiovascular, strength, and flexibility training. The basic kettlebell movements, such as the clean and jerk, help to engage muscles in the entire body all at once. In doing this, kettlebell exercises can often imitate everyday "real world" activities better than other exercises. The exercises and circuits in this book are designed to target all areas of the body.

By increasing repetitions and/or duration, kettlebell exercises will not only build strength, but also build muscular endurance. As mentioned above, kettlebell exercises by their very nature provide a total body workout. They work multiple muscle groups simultaneously and can be repeated continuously for several minutes with or without short breaks. This combination makes the exercises and circuits in this book moderately aerobic in nature and more similar to **high-intensity interval training (HIIT)** than traditional weight training.

Simply put, compared to gym machines and bench exercises, kettlebells make you work harder for each rep. They provide a great combination of strength, flexibility and endurance training.

TIPS ON TECHNIQUE

Like most things in life, technique with kettlebells is everything. The movements used in kettlebell exercises can be hazardous to those with back or shoulder problems as well as those with weak core strength. This is all the more reason to pay extra attention to technique. If carried out correctly, kettlebell training can be as effective, or more effective, than any other type of resistance training when it comes to improving mobility, range of motion, endurance, and strength.

Due to its unbalanced design, beginners to kettlebell training can easily injure themselves. Please take care at all times to perform each exercise with the correct technique and use a weight load or weight loads that suit your ability. It is far better to start out with light weight loads and good form than with heavy weight loads and poor form.

Remember: Bad Technique = Increased Chance of Injury

Five tips to ensure correct form and technique:

1. **Maintain a neutral spine position**: Neutral spine position means that you maintain the normal curves of your entire spine during all exercises.

2. **Keep your grip in a neutral position so your wrist neither flexes nor extends**: Maintaining a strong grip on the kettlebell handle means you are less likely to move your wrist and cause an injury. The bottom of your thumb joint should be in alignment with your wrist when lifting and swinging.

3. **Your center of gravity should be your abdominal area**: When doing kettlebell exercises that require balance, always keep your center of gravity close to the center of your body. It can be easy to lose your balance and injure yourself if you don't.

4. **Drive through with your legs and hips when lifting the kettlebell from a low position to a high position**: When you swing or lift the kettlebell, driving the legs and hips can generate momentum, which allows you to lift heavy weight loads while maintaining good form. Drive your legs and hips by pushing against the floor and pushing your buttocks and hips forward at the same time.

5. **Do not train your muscles to failure**: Due to the dynamic nature of kettlebell exercises, they do not lend themselves well to training to muscle failure. When you push yourself to muscle failure, your form will inevitably suffer and you dramatically increase your chances of getting injured.

WARMING UP & COOLING DOWN

Warming up and cooling down are essential parts of any resistance training program. They help prepare your body for a strenuous workout and help to reduce injury and soreness. It is strongly advised that you begin every workout with some form of warm-up routine and conclude every workout with some form of cool-down routine.

WARMING UP

The basic idea behind "warming up" is to prepare your body, particularly your muscles, for physical activity. A warm-up is therefore performed directly before exercise and generally involves some kind of low-intensity activity to increase blood flow to your muscles. **Jogging is an ideal warm up** as it increases your heart rate and generally prepares you for the more intense physical activity that is to follow. A mild form of stretching can also be helpful as part of a warm-up routine.

THREE-POINT GUIDELINE TO WARMING UP

1. Spend about five minutes warming up. Don't warm up for long periods before dynamic exercise (such as kettlebell training).

2. Address the areas of your body that you are about to exercise.

3. Concentrate on any muscles that feel tight, although if you are injured don't exercise at all!

COOLING DOWN

"Cooling down" is the period straight after exercise when you gradually change from a state of physical exertion to a state of near rest. Just as warming up before exercising is a good idea, it is a good idea to cool down after exercising.

Cooling down has been shown to help remove
lactic acid from the muscles.

Light jogging for about five minutes is again ideal, slowly decreasing the intensity as you go. You will want to rehydrate yourself during the cooling-down period or directly afterwards. As with warming up, feel free to include some light stretching as part of your cool-down routine.

THE PROGRAMS

This book contains nine different kettlebell workout programs, each designed for a different purpose. All nine programs are to be performed in **circuits**, which means you will perform one set of each exercise in the program consecutively without rest between sets. After you have completed one full circuit, you will rest for the predetermined time listed for of each program before beginning the next circuit.

EASY TOTAL BODY STRENGTH CIRCUIT

This circuit is ideal for beginners looking to improve their strength and aerobic fitness.

EQUIPMENT REQUIRED: Two kettlebells of equal weight.

INSTRUCTIONS: Complete the circuit below **3 times with 2 minutes rest** between circuits.

Vary the kettlebell weight according to your ability and fitness level.

EXERCISES:

- Alternating Bicep Curls

- Shoulder Press

- Russian Twists

- Full Extension Sit-ups

- Dead Lifts

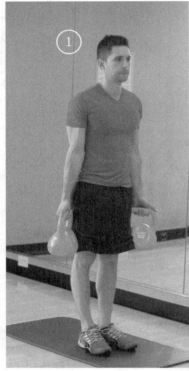

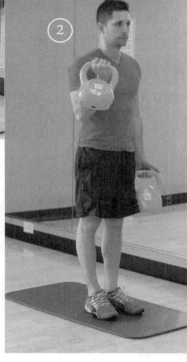

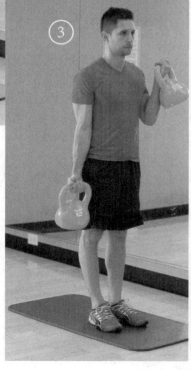

ALTERNATING BICEP CURLS

REPS: 5

DESCRIPTION/NOTES: Stand holding one kettlebell in each hand with your arms hanging at your sides. Alternately curl each kettlebell up to your shoulder before returning to the starting position and repeating with your other arm.

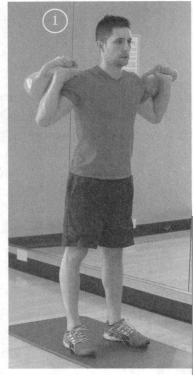

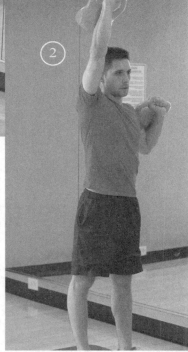

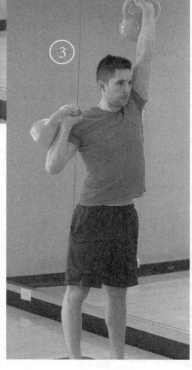

SHOULDER PRESS

REPS: 5

DESCRIPTION/NOTES: Stand holding one kettlebell in each hand at shoulder height in the "rack" position (see photo 1). Alternately press each kettlebell up above your head until your arm is fully extended. Return your arm to the starting position in a controlled manner and repeat with your other arm.

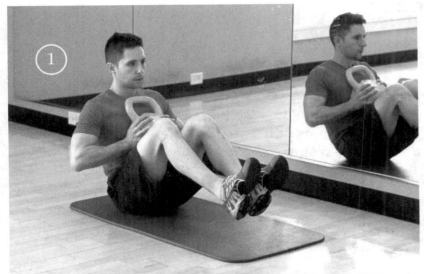

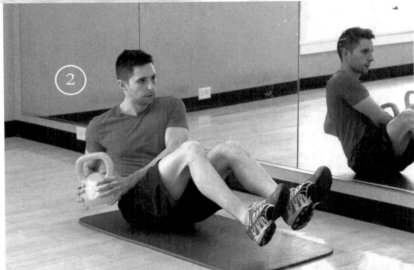

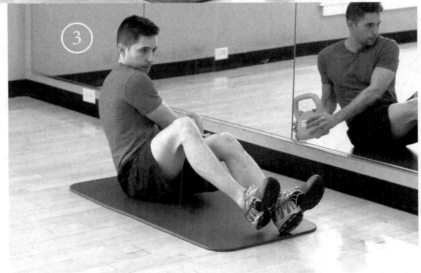

RUSSIAN TWISTS

REPS: 10

DESCRIPTION/NOTES: Sit with your legs bent at the knees and hold one kettlebell in front of your chest with both hands. Twist your torso to the left and allow your arms to extend so that the kettlebell is balanced just above the floor on your left side. Then twist your torso to the right and bring the kettlebell so that it is balanced just above the floor on your right side.

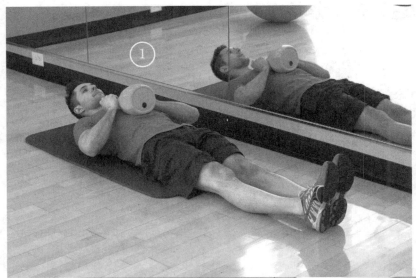

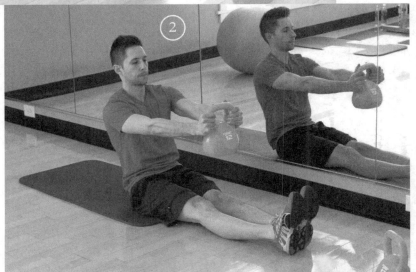

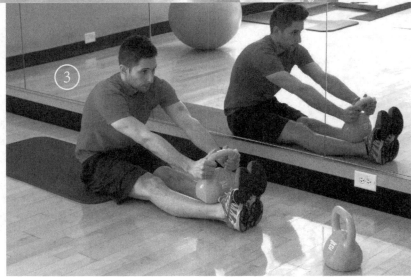

FULL EXTENSION SIT-UPS

REPS: 10

DESCRIPTION/NOTES: Lie on your back with your legs extended and hold one kettlebell in both hands close to your chest. Sit up and fully extend your arms in front of you. Reach forward to touch your feet with the kettlebell. Return to the starting position in a controlled manner and repeat.

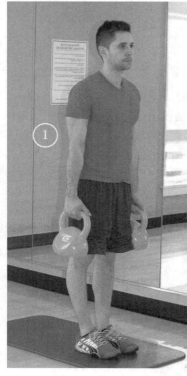

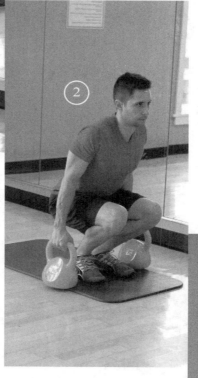

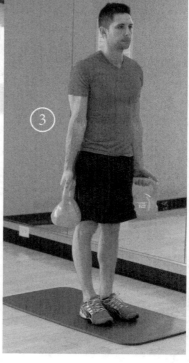

DEAD LIFTS

REPS: 10

DESCRIPTION/NOTES: Stand holding one kettlebell in each hand with your arms at your sides. Keep your back straight and your feet flat on the floor as you bend your legs to squat down. The kettlebells should graze the floor before you stand back up into the starting position.

INTERMEDIATE TOTAL BODY STRENGTH CIRCUIT

This circuit is great for those with a reasonable level of fitness looking to improve their strength.

EQUIPMENT REQUIRED: Two kettlebells of equal weight.

INSTRUCTIONS: Complete the circuit below **3 times with 90 seconds rest** between circuits.

Vary the kettlebell weight according to your ability and fitness level.

EXERCISES:

- Single-Arm Clean & Press

- Kettlebell Swings

- Single Leg "V" Sit-ups

- Double Kettlebell Sit-ups

- Same-Leg Lunges

- Squats

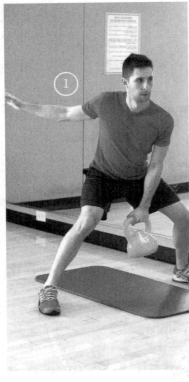

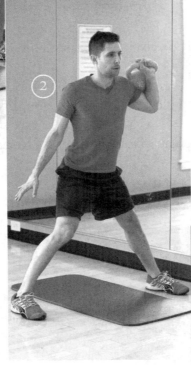

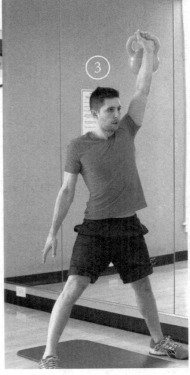

SINGLE-ARM CLEAN & PRESS

REPS: 10

DESCRIPTION/NOTES: Stand with your knees bent and hold one kettlebell in your left hand between your legs. Your off hand should be used for balance throughout this exercise. Thrust upwards, bringing the kettlebell towards your right shoulder and assume the "rack" position (see photo 2) with your knees still bent. From here, in one fluid motion stand straight up and press the kettlebell above your shoulder, extending your arm upwards. Return the kettlebell to the starting position in a controlled manner. Once you have completed the desired number of repetitions, switch to your right hand.

KETTLEBELL SWINGS

REPS: 10

DESCRIPTION/NOTES: Stand with your knees bent and hold one kettlebell in both hands between your legs. While keeping your back straight and your feet flat on the floor, thrust upwards, swinging the kettlebell straight out in front of you with both arms fully extended. Swing your arms back down and return to the starting position in a controlled manner. Repeat.

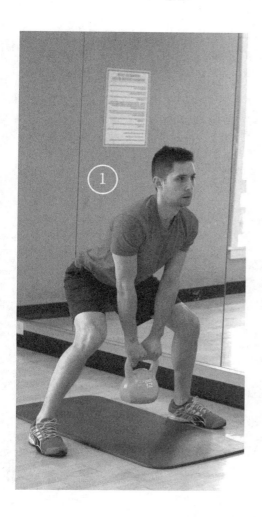

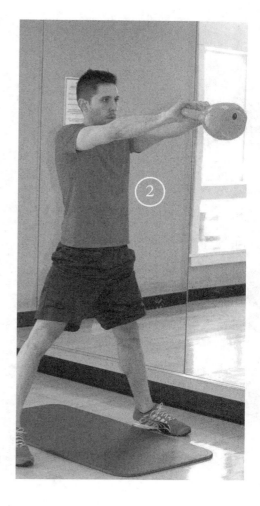

SINGLE LEG "V" SIT-UPS

REPS: 5 REPS FOR EACH LEG

DESCRIPTION/NOTES: Lie on your back with your legs extended and hold one kettlebell in both hands behind your head with your arms fully extended. Sit up with your arms still fully extended and simultaneously raise your right leg off the floor. Bring the kettlebell towards your raised foot so that your body forms a "V" shape. Return to the starting position in a controlled manner and repeat with the same leg for the desired number of reps and then repeat with the other leg.

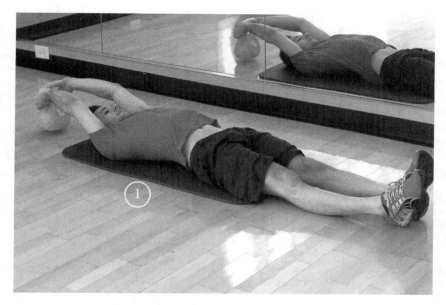

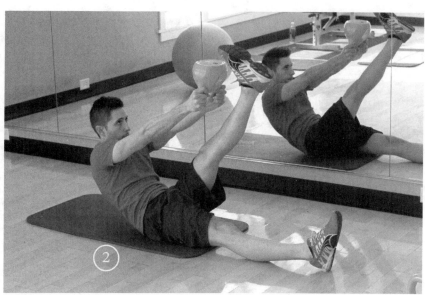

DOUBLE KETTLEBELL SIT-UPS

REPS: 10

DESCRIPTION/NOTES: Lie on your back with your legs extended and hold two kettlebells close to your chest. Sit up, keeping both kettlebells by your chest. Your legs should be slightly bent with your feet flat on the floor. Return to the starting position and repeat.

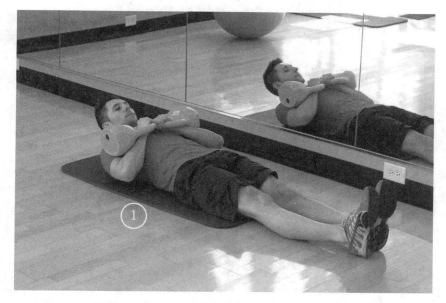

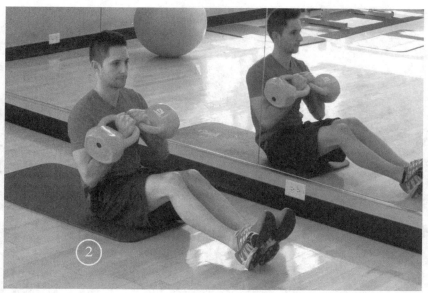

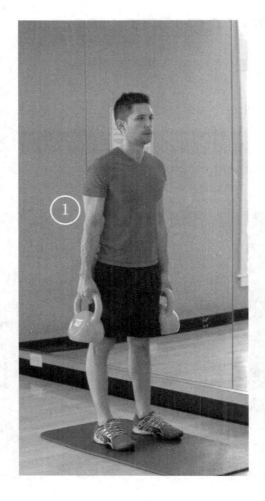

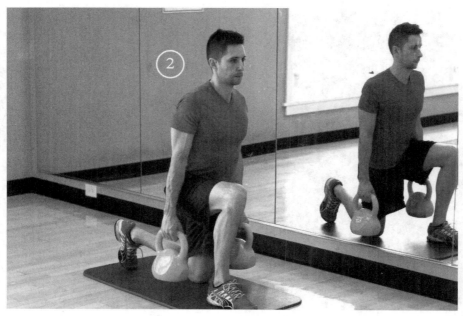

SAME-LEG LUNGES

REPS: 10 REPS FOR EACH LEG

DESCRIPTION/NOTES: Stand holding one kettlebell in each hand at your sides. Lunge forward with your right leg so that your left knee is bent just above the floor. Keep your back straight and the kettlebells balanced by your sides. Push off your right leg in order to return to the starting position. Once you have completed the desired number of repetitions with your right leg, switch to your left.

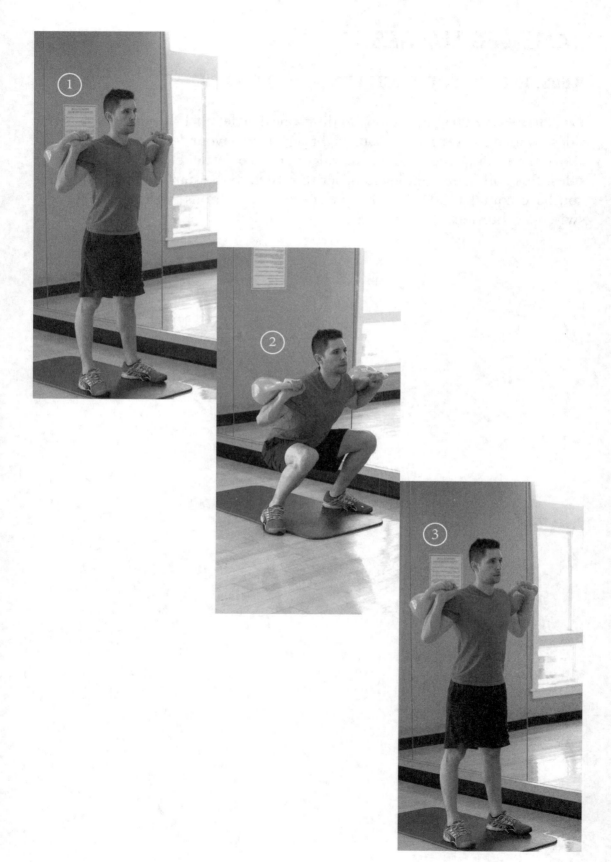

SQUATS

REPS: 10

DESCRIPTION/NOTES: Stand holding one kettlebell in each hand by your shoulders in the "rack" position. Bend your knees at a 90 degree angle keeping your back straight and your knees in line with your feet. Stand up to return to the starting position and repeat.

HARDCORE TOTAL BODY STRENGTH CIRCUIT

This circuit is ideal for those with a good level of fitness, who love high-intensity interval training (HIIT).

EQUIPMENT REQUIRED: Two kettlebells of equal weight.

INSTRUCTIONS: Complete the circuit below **3 times.** Take a **1 minute** rest between circuits.

Vary the kettlebell weight according to your ability and fitness level.

EXERCISES:

- Shoulder Flyes
- Dynamic Push-ups
- Burpees
- Under Leg Sit-ups
- Double Kettlebell Swings
- Get-ups

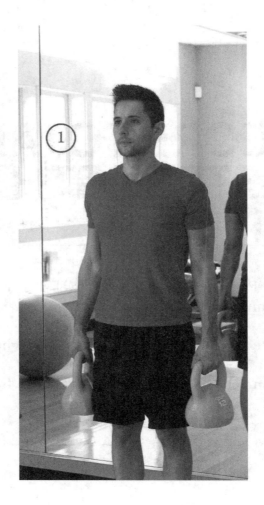

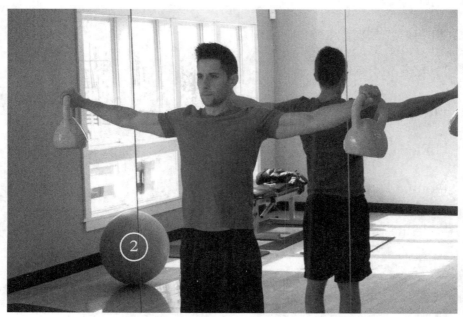

SHOULDER FLYES

REPS: 10

DESCRIPTION/NOTES: Stand holding one kettlebell in each hand at your sides. Keep your arms as straight as possible and raise them laterally until they are parallel with the floor. Lower your arms in a controlled manner to return to the starting position and repeat.

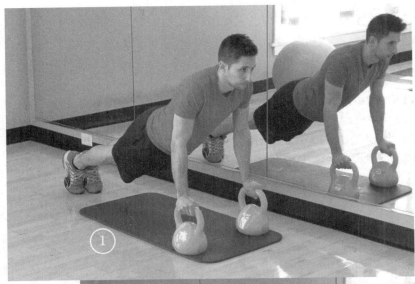

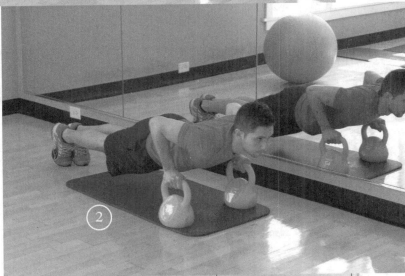

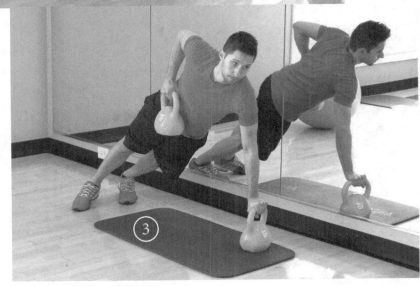

DYNAMIC PUSH-UPS

REPS: 10

DESCRIPTION/NOTES: Lie in the push-up position with a kettlebell in each hand. With your weight on the kettlebells, perform a standard push-up (down and up) and then bring one kettlebell off the floor towards your chest in a rowing motion. Lower the kettlebell back to the floor and repeat with the other hand. Return to the starting position and repeat.

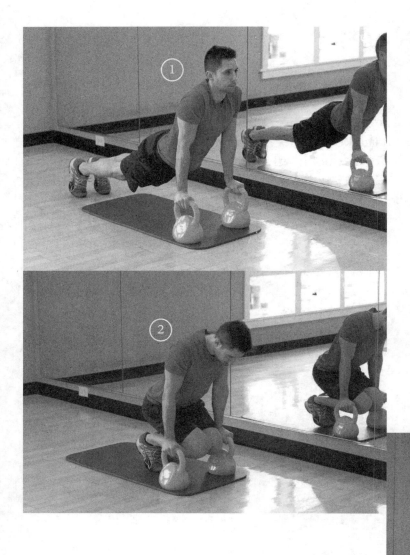

BURPEES

REPS: 10

DESCRIPTION/NOTES: Begin in the push-up position with a kettlebell in each hand. With your weight on the kettlebells, bring your knees and feet up to your chest and, in one fluid motion, spring upwards into the standing position with the kettlebells at your sides. From the standing position, squat back down and place both kettlebells on the floor, then thrust your legs out behind you back into the original push-up position.

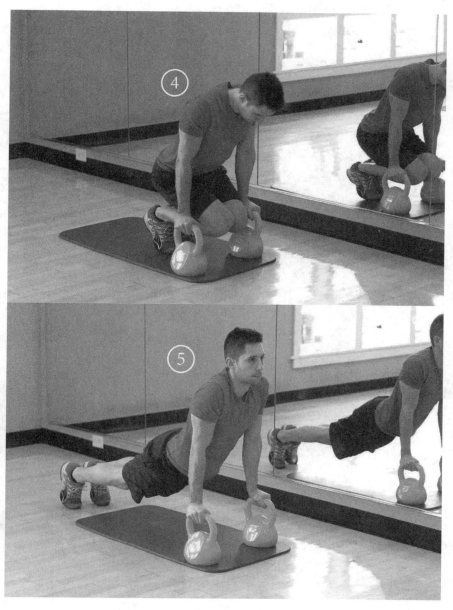

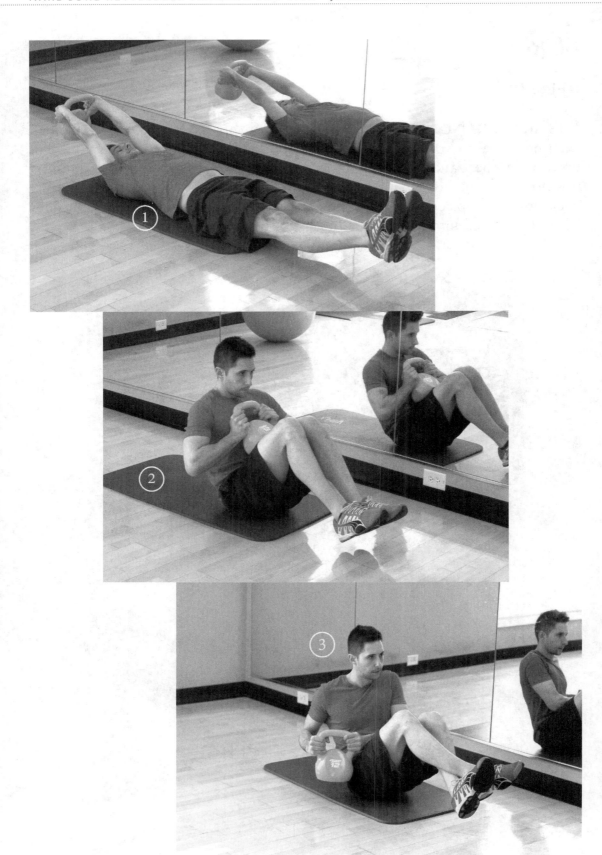

UNDER LEG SIT-UPS

REPS: 5 REPS IN EACH DIRECTION

DESCRIPTION/NOTES: Lie on your back with your legs extended and hold one kettlebell in both hands above your head. Sit up and bring the kettlebell to your chest while simultaneously bringing you knees into your chest. Balance in this seated position and pass the kettlebell under your legs from one hand to the other. Return to the starting position and repeat.

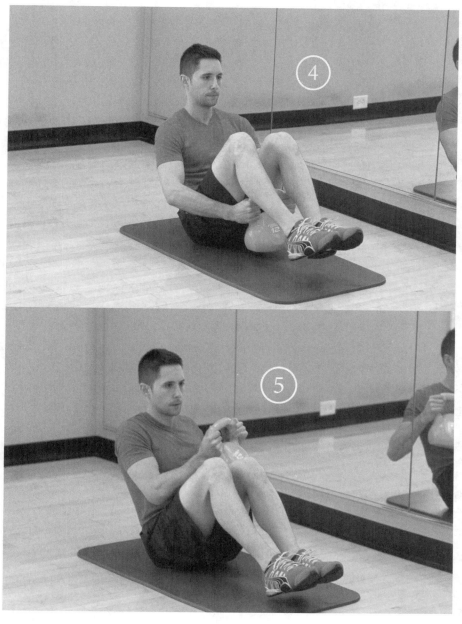

DOUBLE KETTLEBELL SWINGS

REPS: 10

DESCRIPTION/NOTES: Stand with your knees bent and hold one kettlebell in each hand between your legs using an overhand grip. While maintaining a straight back and your feet flat on the floor, thrust upwards, swinging both kettlebells up above your head with your arms are fully extended. Swing your arms back down into the starting position in a controlled manner and repeat.

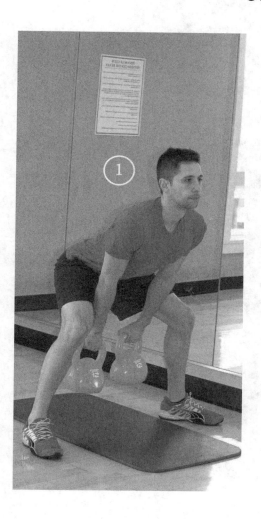

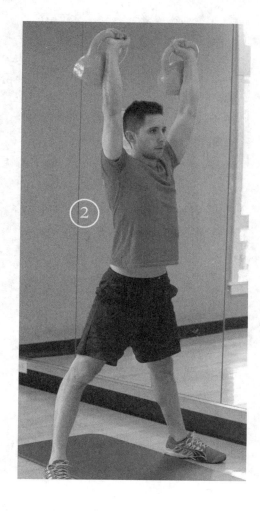

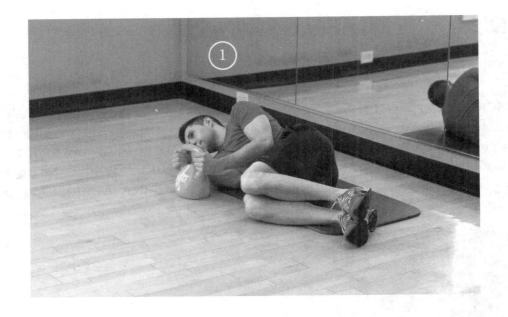

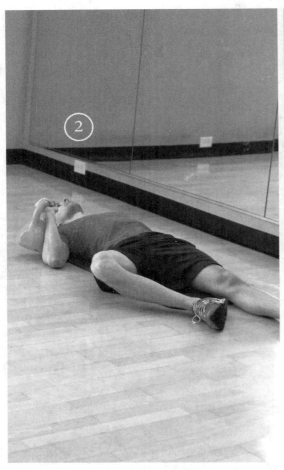

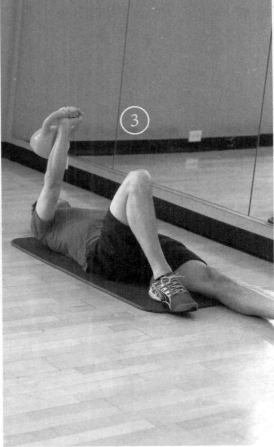

GET-UPS

REPS: 5 REPS ON EACH SIDE

DESCRIPTION/NOTES: Lie on your side in the fetal position and hold one kettlebell with both hands. Roll onto your back with the kettlebell now in one hand. Fully extend the kettlebell above your chest with one leg bent as you prepare to stand up. With the assistance of your off-hand pushing against the floor, begin to stand up with the kettlebell held above your head. Once you are standing upright with your arm full extended above your head, you will want to reverse the process to get back into the starting position to repeat.

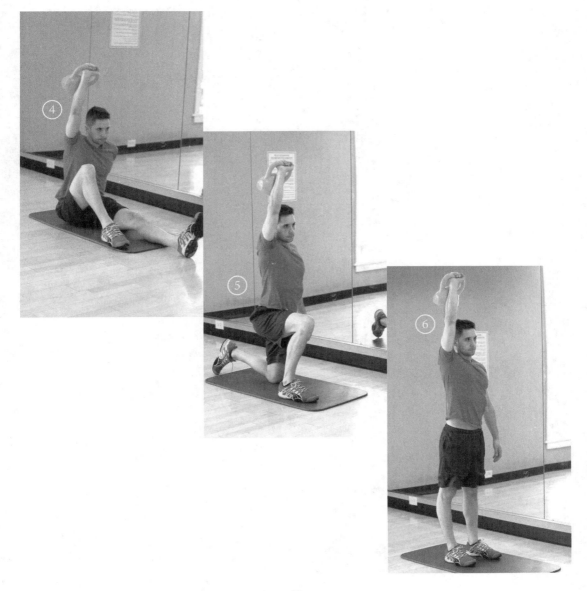

UPPER BODY CONDITIONING CIRCUIT

This circuit is great for those with a reasonable level of fitness looking to improve their upper body strength.

EQUIPMENT REQUIRED: Two kettlebells of equal weight.

INSTRUCTIONS: Complete the circuit below **3 times.** Take a **2 minute** rest between circuits.

Vary the kettlebell weight according to your ability and fitness level.

EXERCISES:

- Shoulder Rotations

- Push-out, Push-ups

- Lightning Bolt

- Overhead Triceps Extensions

- Dynamic Push-ups

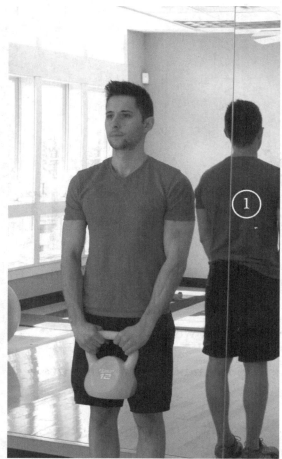

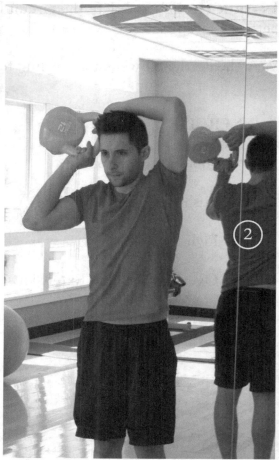

SHOULDER ROTATIONS

REPS: 10 REPS IN EACH DIRECTION

DESCRIPTION/NOTES: Stand holding one kettlebell in both hands in front of you at your waist. In one fluid motion, swing the kettlebell up and to the left, behind your head, and back down to the starting position. Repeat for the desired number of repetitions.

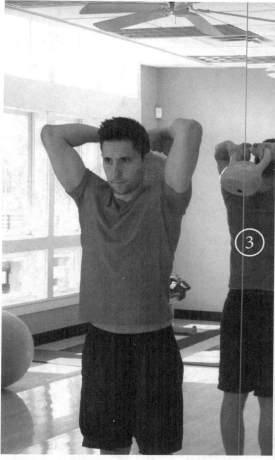

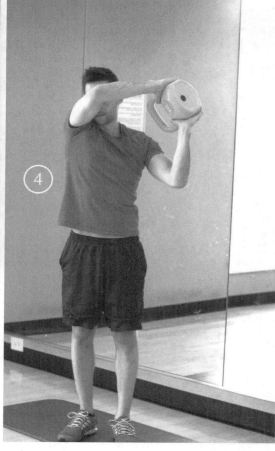

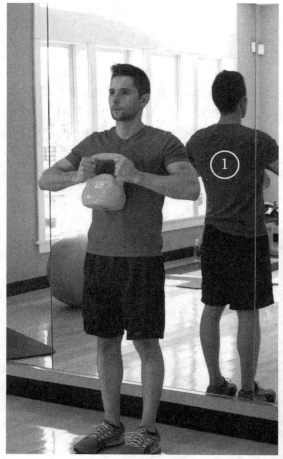

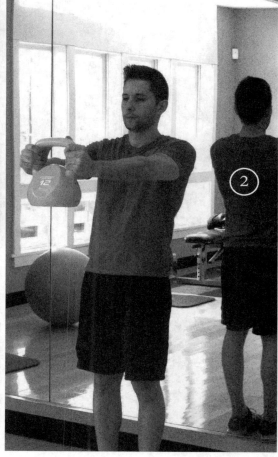

PUSH-OUT, PUSH-UPS

REPS: 10

DESCRIPTION/NOTES: Stand holding one kettlebell in both hands in front of you at chest height. Extend your arms forward with the kettlebell. Bring the kettlebell back to your chest and then extend your arms upward over your head. Bring the kettlebell back to the starting position in a controlled manner and repeat.

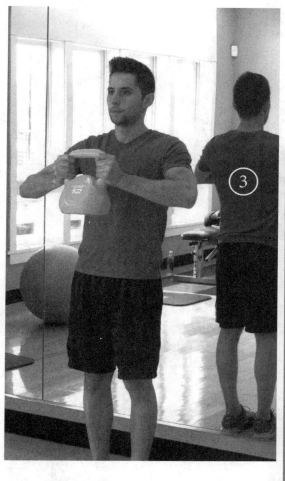

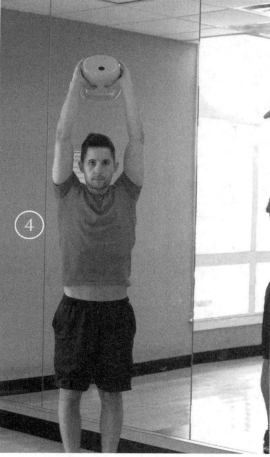

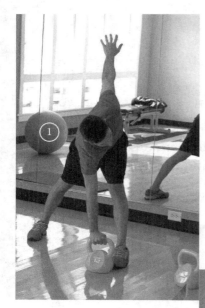

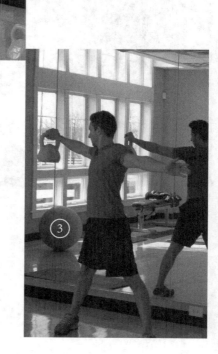

LIGHTNING BOLT

REPS: 10 REPS FOR EACH HAND

DESCRIPTION/NOTES: Stand with your legs shoulder width apart, holding one kettlebell with your right hand in front of your left foot. Your left arm should be used for balance during this exercise. Thrust upwards, bringing the kettlebell to your right shoulder into the "rack" position, then, in one fluid motion, thrust your right arm out to your side, extending at a 45 degree angle. Bring the kettlebell back down to your left foot in a controlled manner and repeat.

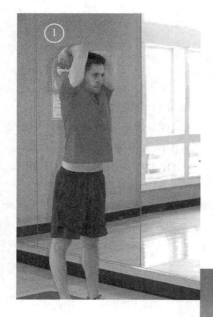

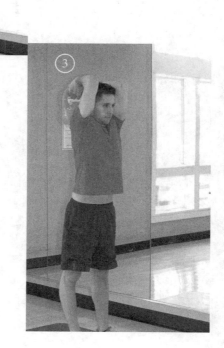

OVERHEAD TRICEPS EXTENSIONS

REPS: 10

DESCRIPTION/NOTES: Stand holding one kettlebell in both hands behind your head with your elbows bent and tucked in close to your head. Extend your arms upwards, bringing the kettlebell above your head. Return under control and repeat.

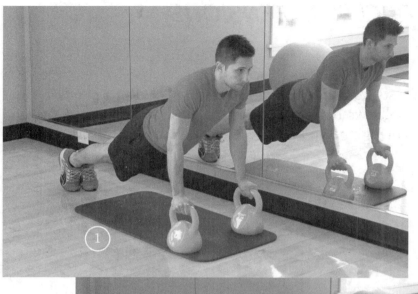

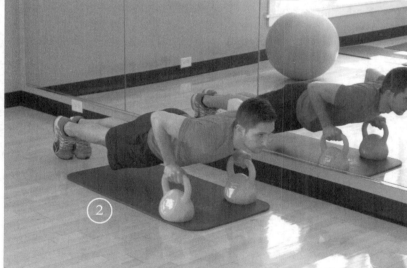

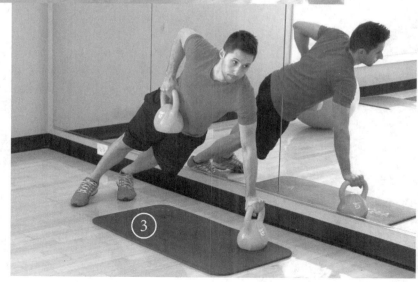

DYNAMIC PUSH-UPS

REPS: 5 REPS FOR EACH HAND

DESCRIPTION/NOTES: Lie in the push-up position with a kettlebell in each hand. With your weight on the kettlebells, perform a standard push-up (down and up) and then bring one kettlebell off the floor towards your chest in a rowing motion. Lower the kettlebell back to the floor and repeat with the other hand. Return to the starting position and repeat.

ABDOMINALS & CORE CONDITIONING CIRCUIT

This circuit is great for those with a reasonable level of fitness looking to improve their abdominal and core body strength.

EQUIPMENT REQUIRED: Two kettlebells of equal weight.

INSTRUCTIONS: Complete the circuit below **3 times.** Take a **2 minute** rest between circuits.

Vary the kettlebell weight according to your ability and fitness level.

EXERCISES:

- Russian Twists

- Horizontal Wood Chops

- Straight Arm Sit-ups

- Figure 8's

- Sit-up & Punch-outs

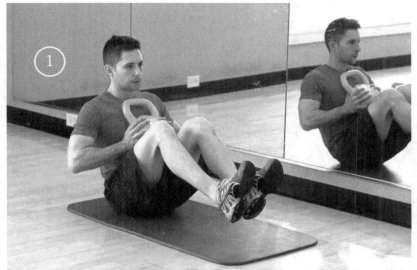

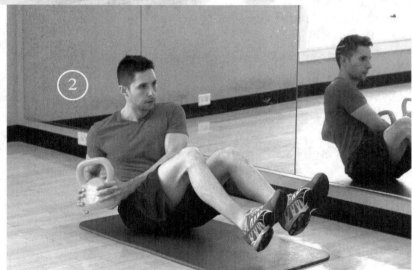

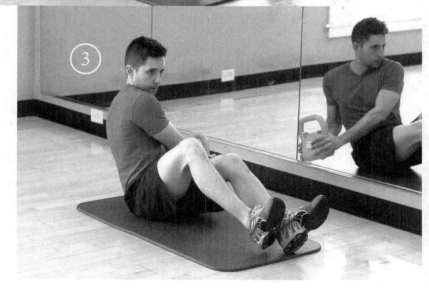

RUSSIAN TWISTS

REPS: 10

DESCRIPTION/NOTES: Sit with your legs bent at the knees and hold one kettlebell in front of your chest with both hands. Twist your torso to the left and allow your arms to extend so that the kettlebell is balanced just above the floor on your left side. Then twist your torso to the right and bring the kettlebell so that it is balanced just above the floor on your right side.

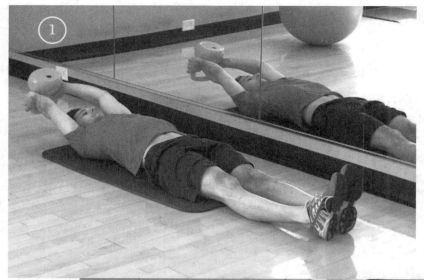

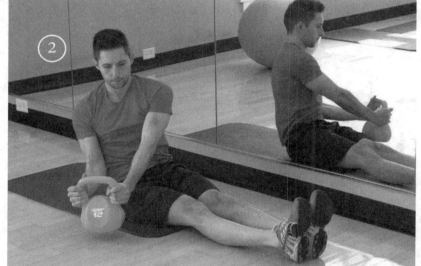

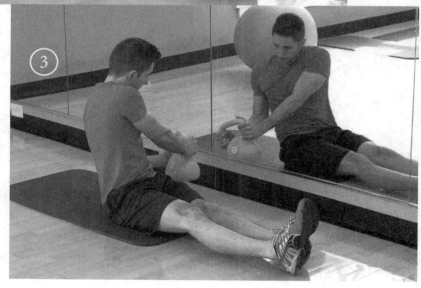

HORIZONTAL WOOD CHOPS

REPS: 5 REPS ON EACH SIDE

DESCRIPTION/NOTES: Lie on your back with your legs extended and hold one kettlebell in both hands with your arms extended behind your head. With your arms remaining fully extended, sit up and bring the kettlebell over your head and down to the right side of your body. Return to the starting position and repeat to the left side of your body. Repeat for the desired number of repetitions.

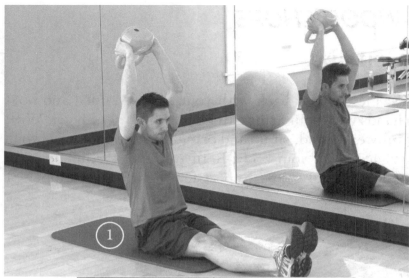

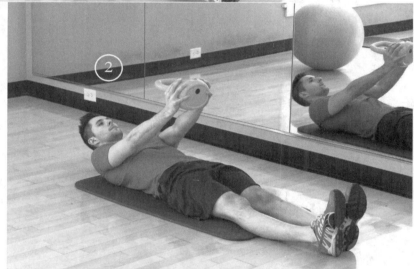

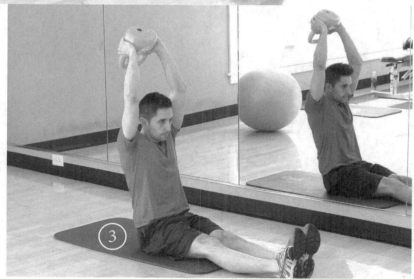

STRAIGHT ARM SIT-UPS

REPS: 10

DESCRIPTION/NOTES: Sit upright on the floor with your legs extended and hold one kettlebell in both hands above your head with your arms extended. Keeping your arms extended, lie down until your back is flat on the floor and the kettlebell is above your chest forming a 90 degree angle. Sit back up to return to the starting position and repeat.

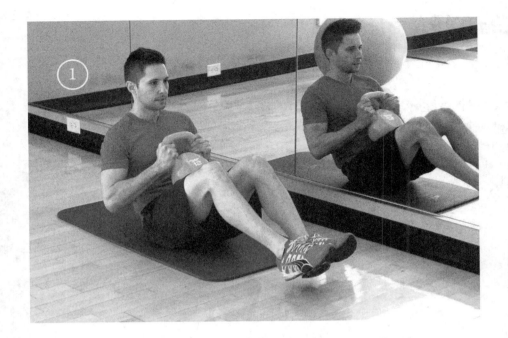

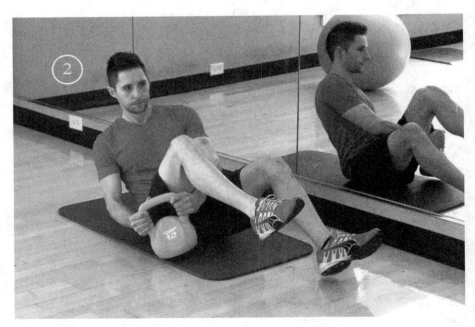

FIGURE 8'S

REPS: 10

DESCRIPTION/NOTES: Sit on the floor with your legs bent at the knees and your feet off the floor. Hold one kettlebell in front of your chest with both hands. Keeping your feet off the floor, pass the kettlebell from one hand to the other under one leg, over the other leg, and then back under the second leg and over the first leg so that you are performing a "figure 8" with the kettlebell. Return to the starting position and repeat.

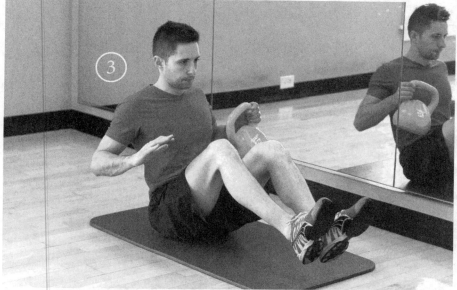

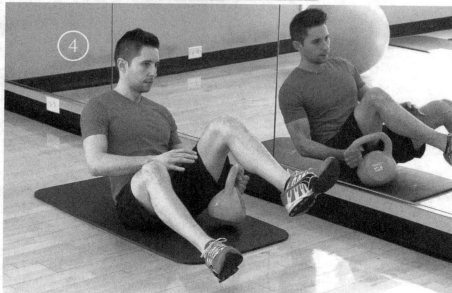

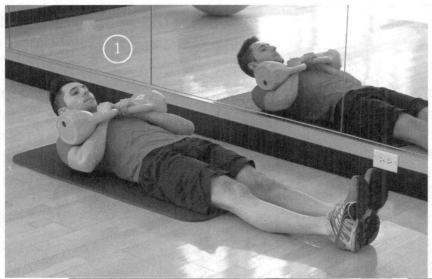

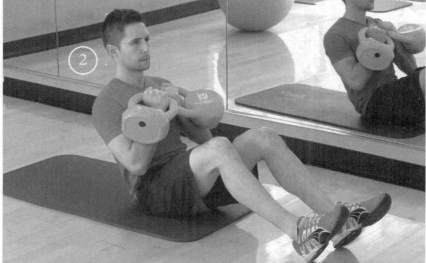

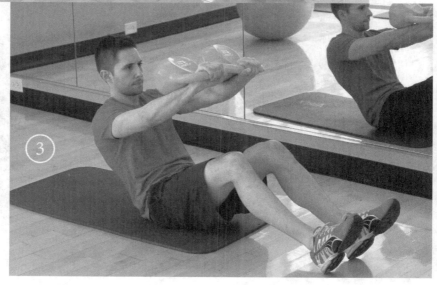

SIT-UP & PUNCH-OUTS

REPS: 10

DESCRIPTION/NOTES: Lie on your back with your legs extended and bent at the knees. Hold a kettlebell in each hand by your shoulders. Perform a sit up and push both kettlebells out in front of you until your arms are fully extended. Return to the start position in a controlled manner and repeat.

LEG CONDITIONING CIRCUIT

This circuit is great for those with a reasonable level of fitness looking to improve their lower body strength.

EQUIPMENT REQUIRED: Two kettlebells of equal weight.

INSTRUCTIONS: Complete the circuit below **3 times.** Take a **2 minute** rest between circuits.

Vary the kettlebell weight according to your ability and fitness level.

EXERCISES:

- Overhead Squats

- Dynamic Jump Lunges

- Burpees

- Side Lunges

- Double Kettlebell Clean

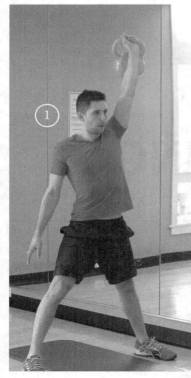

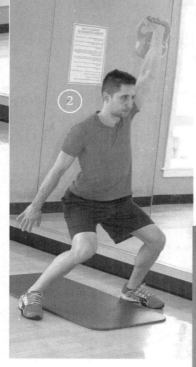

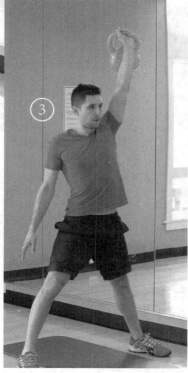

OVERHEAD SQUATS

REPS: 5 REPS FOR EACH LEG

DESCRIPTION/NOTES: Stand holding one kettlebell in your right hand above your head with your arm fully extended. While keeping your arm fully extended, bend your knees to a 90 degree angle. Still keeping the kettlebell over your head, return to the starting position and repeat.

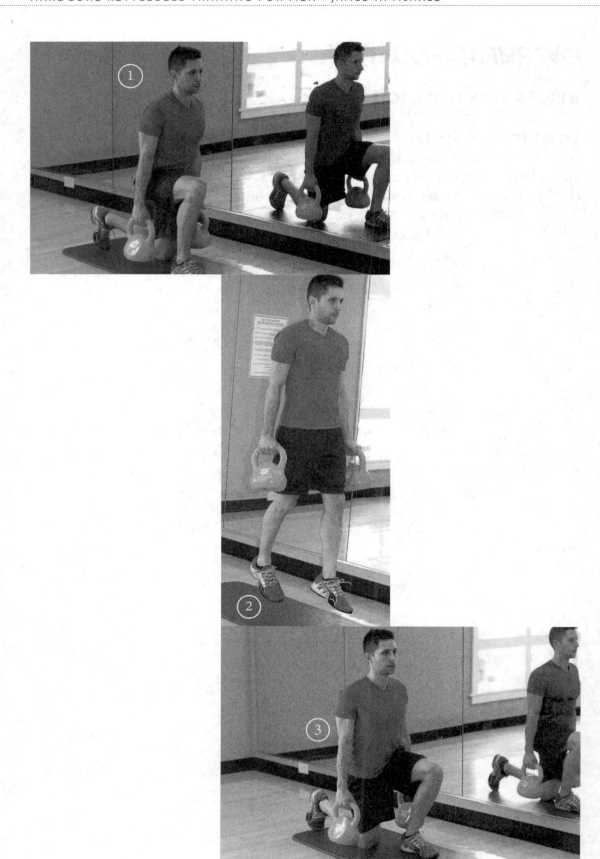

DYNAMIC JUMP LUNGES

REPS: 5 REPS FOR EACH LEG

DESCRIPTION/NOTES: Stand in the lunge position with one leg in front of you, bent at the knee, and the other leg behind you and hold a kettlebell in each hand with your arms at your sides. Spring upwards and jump off the floor. While in the air, switch the position of your legs and land in the lunge position with the other leg in front of you. Repeat for the desired number of repetitions.

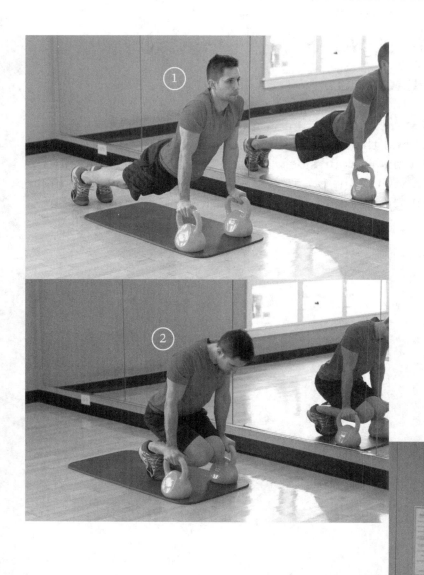

BURPEES

REPS: 10 REPS FOR EACH LEG

DESCRIPTION/NOTES: Begin in the push-up position with a kettlebell in each hand. With your weight on the kettlebells, bring your knees and feet up to your chest and, in one fluid motion, spring upwards into the standing position with the kettlebells at your sides. From the standing position, squat back down and place both kettlebells on the floor, then thrust your legs out behind you back into the original push-up position.

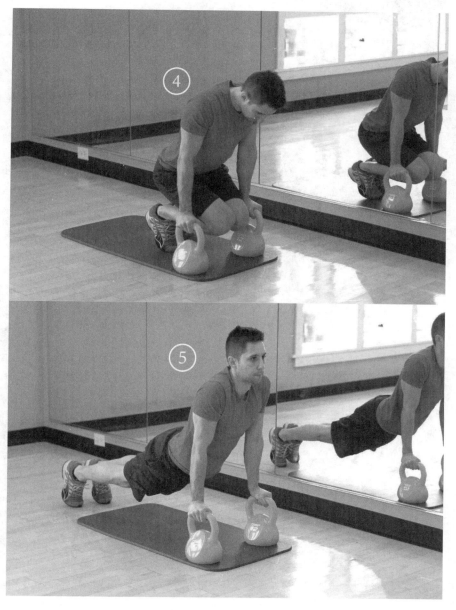

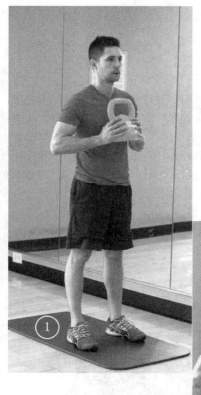

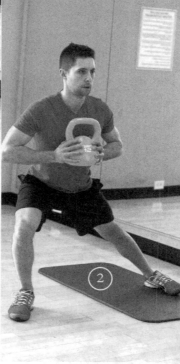

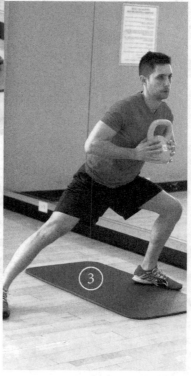

SIDE LUNGES

REPS: 5 REPS FOR EACH LEG

DESCRIPTION/NOTES: Stand holding one kettlebell close to your chest. Take a large step to your right, bending your right knee and keeping your back straight. Make sure your foot and knee are aligned so as not to put too much pressure on your knee. Pushing off your right foot, spring back to the starting position and repeat to your left side.

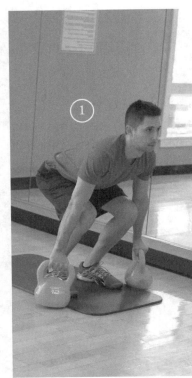

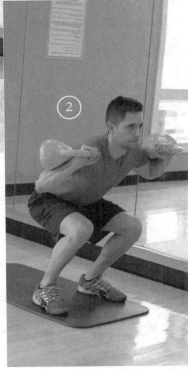

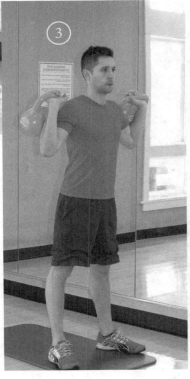

DOUBLE KETTLEBELL CLEAN

REPS: 10 REPS FOR EACH LEG

DESCRIPTION/NOTES: Stand with your knees bent and grip a kettlebell in each hand on the ground using an overhand grip. Thrust upwards, using your hips to swing the kettlebells up to your shoulders (i.e. the "rack" position – see photo 2). While swinging the kettlebells up to your shoulders, bend your knees and "sit" into the squat position. In one fluid motion push-upwards into a standing position with the kettlebells still in the "rack" position. Return the kettlebells to the floor in a controlled manner and repeat.

EASY FAT BURNING CIRCUIT

This circuit is ideal for beginners looking to burn fat and improve their aerobic fitness.

EQUIPMENT REQUIRED: Two kettlebells of equal weight.

INSTRUCTIONS: Complete the circuit below **5 times.** Take a **2 minutes** rest between circuits.

Vary the kettlebell weight according to your ability and fitness level.

EXERCISES:

- Kettlebell Swings

- Dynamic Push-ups

- Single-Arm Kettlebell Swings

- Squats

KETTLEBELL SWINGS

REPS: 20

DESCRIPTION/NOTES: Stand with your knees bent and hold one kettlebell in both hands between your legs. While keeping your back straight and your feet flat on the floor, thrust upwards, swinging the kettlebell straight out in front of you with both arms fully extended. Swing your arms back down and return to the starting position in a controlled manner. Repeat.

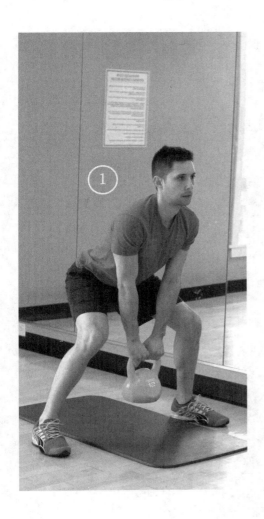

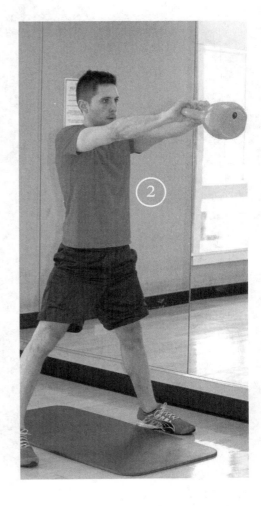

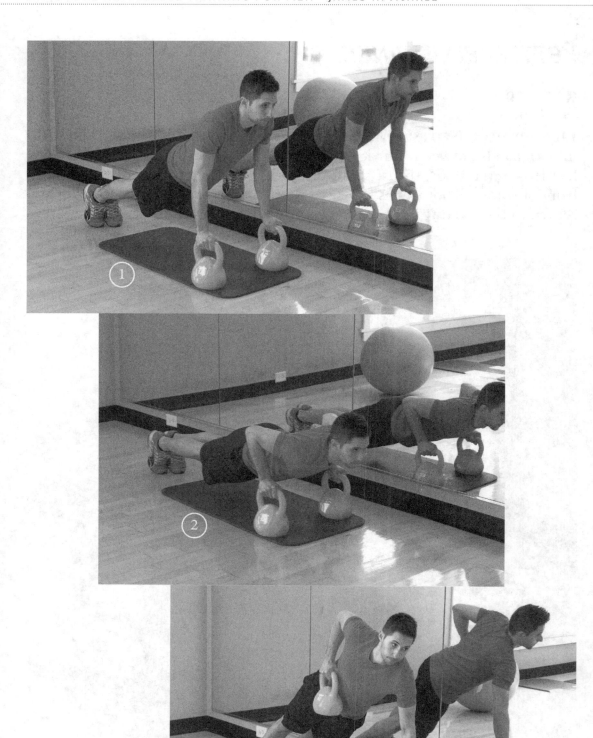

DYNAMIC PUSH-UPS

REPS: 10

DESCRIPTION/NOTES: Begin in the push-up position with a kettlebell in each hand. With your weight on the kettlebells, perform a standard push-up (down and up) and then bring one kettlebell off the floor towards your chest in a rowing motion. Lower the kettlebell back to the floor and repeat with the other hand. Return to the starting position and repeat.

SINGLE-ARM KETTLEBELL SWINGS

REPS: 10 REPS FOR EACH ARM

DESCRIPTION/NOTES: Stand with your knees bent and hold one kettlebell in your left hand between your legs. Your off hand should be used for balance throughout this exercise. While keeping your back straight and your feet flat on the floor, thrust upwards, swinging the kettlebell straight out in front of you with your arm fully extended. Swing your arm back down and return to the starting position in a controlled manner. Once you have completed the desired number of repetitions, switch to your right hand.

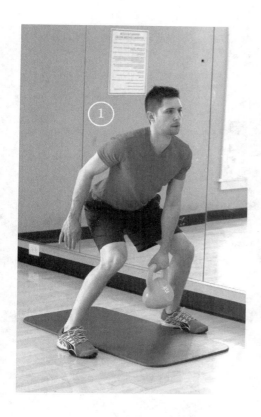

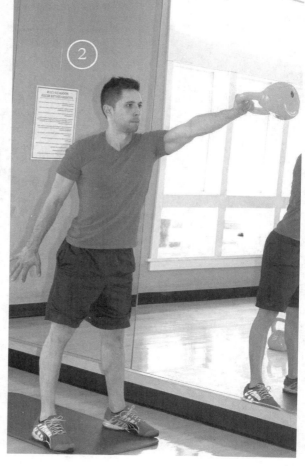

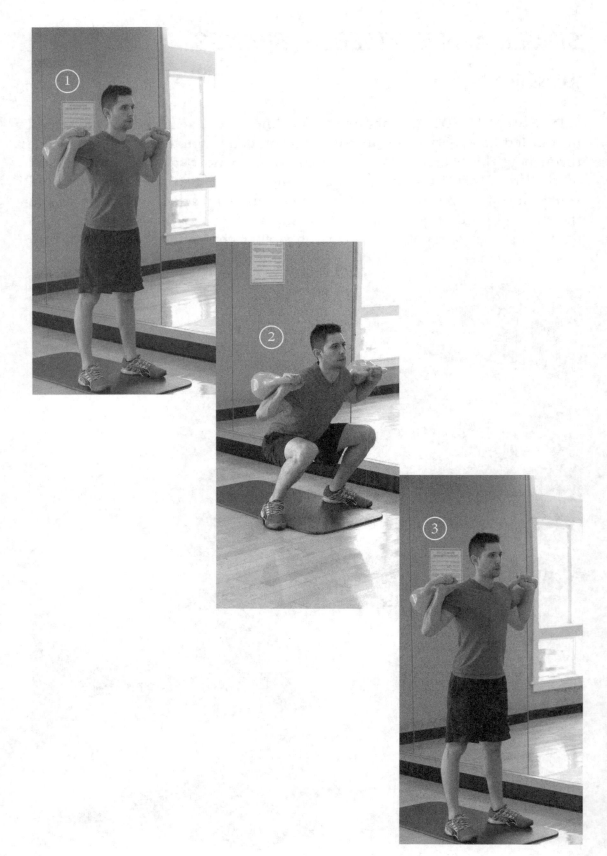

SQUATS

REPS: 20

DESCRIPTION/NOTES: Stand holding one kettlebell in each hand by your shoulders in the "rack" position. Bend your knees at a 90 degree angle keeping your back straight and your knees in line with your feet. Stand up to return to the starting position and repeat.

INTERMEDIATE FAT BURNING CIRCUIT

This circuit is great for those with a reasonable level of fitness looking to burn fat and improve their aerobic fitness.

EQUIPMENT REQUIRED: Two kettlebells of equal weight.

INSTRUCTIONS: Complete the circuit below **5 times.** Take a **2 minute** rest between circuits.

Vary the kettlebell weight according to your ability and fitness level.

EXERCISES:

- Kettlebell Swings

- Single-Arm Clean & Press

- Burpees

- Snatches

HARDCORE KETTLEBELL TRAINING FOR MEN • *JAMES H. McHALE*

KETTLEBELL SWINGS

REPS: 20

DESCRIPTION/NOTES: Stand with your knees bent and hold one kettlebell in both hands between your legs. While keeping your back straight and your feet flat on the floor, thrust upwards, swinging the kettlebell straight out in front of you with both arms fully extended. Swing your arms back down and return to the starting position in a controlled manner. Repeat.

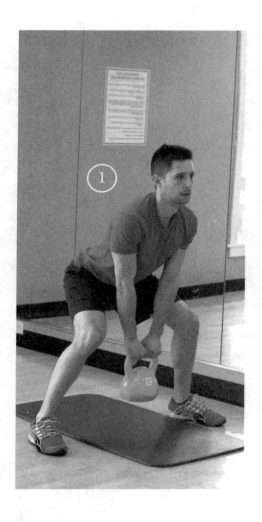

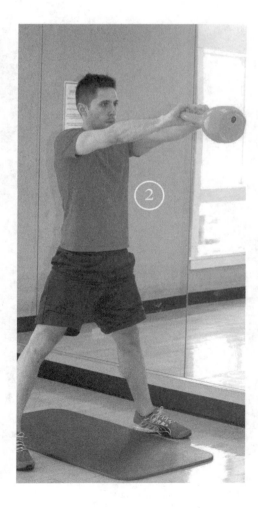

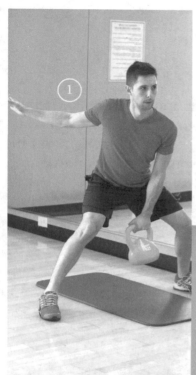

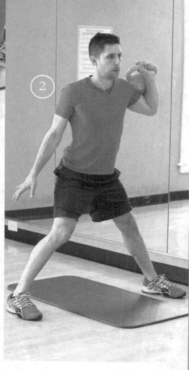

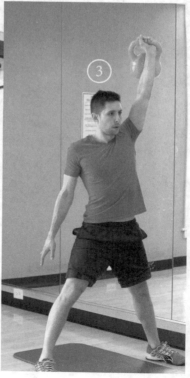

SINGLE-ARM CLEAN & PRESS

REPS: 10 REPS FOR EACH ARM

DESCRIPTION/NOTES: Stand with your knees bent and hold one kettlebell in your left hand between your legs. Your off hand should be used for balance throughout this exercise. Thrust upwards, bringing the kettlebell towards your right shoulder and assume the "rack" position (see photo 2) with your knees still bent. From here, in one fluid motion stand straight up and press the kettlebell above your shoulder, extending your arm upwards. Return the kettlebell to the starting position in a controlled manner. Once you have completed the desired number of repetitions, switch to your right hand.

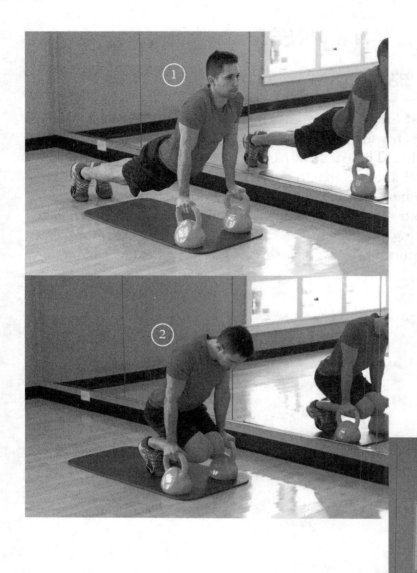

BURPEES

REPS: 20

DESCRIPTION/NOTES: Begin in the push-up position with a kettlebell in each hand. With your weight on the kettlebells, bring your knees and feet up to your chest and, in one fluid motion, spring upwards into the standing position with the kettlebells at your sides. From the standing position, squat back down and place both kettlebells on the floor, then thrust your legs out behind you back into the original push-up position.

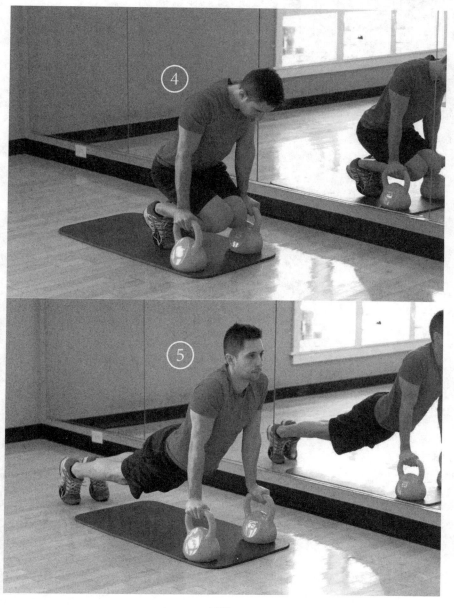

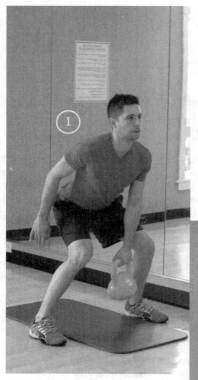

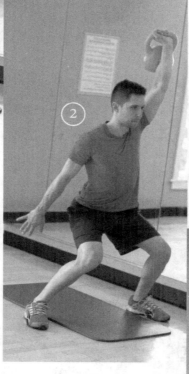

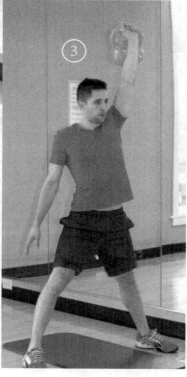

SNATCHES

REPS: 10 REPS FOR EACH ARM

DESCRIPTION/NOTES: Stand with your knees bent and hold one kettlebell in your left hand between your legs. Your off hand should be used for balance throughout this exercise. While keeping your back straight and your feet flat on the floor, thrust upwards, swinging the kettlebell above your head and ensuring the kettlebell is positioned behind your wrist. While thrusting upwards, simultaneously squat down, bending your knees at a 90 degree angle and then stand up fully. In a controlled manner swing your arm back down to the starting position. Once you have completed the desired number of repetitions, switch to your right hand.

HARDCORE FAT BURNING CIRCUIT

This circuit is ideal for those with a good level of fitness, who love HIIT training and want to burn fat.

EQUIPMENT REQUIRED: Two kettlebells of equal weight.

INSTRUCTIONS: Complete the circuit below **5 times.** Take a **2 minute** rest between circuits.

Vary the kettlebell weight according to your ability and fitness level.

EXERCISES:

- Kettlebell Swings

- Overhead Squats

- Burpees

- Get-ups

KETTLEBELL SWINGS

REPS: 20

DESCRIPTION/NOTES: Stand with your knees bent and hold one kettlebell in both hands between your legs. While keeping your back straight and your feet flat on the floor, thrust upwards, swinging the kettlebell straight out in front of you with both arms fully extended. Swing your arms back down and return to the starting position in a controlled manner. Repeat.

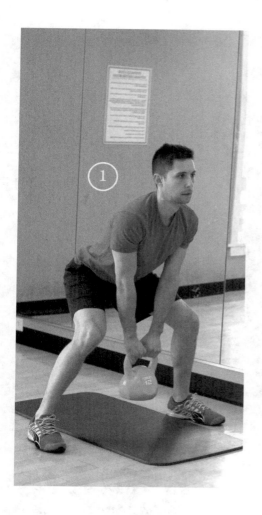

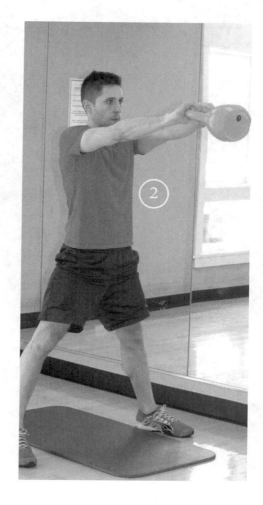

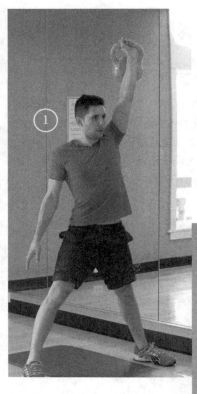

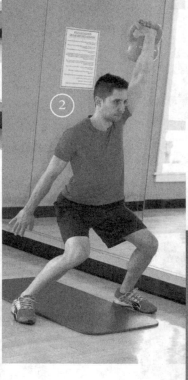

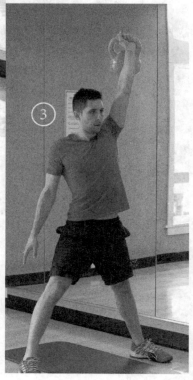

OVERHEAD SQUATS

REPS: 10 REPS FOR EACH ARM

DESCRIPTION/NOTES: Stand holding one kettlebell in your right hand above your head with your arm fully extended. While keeping your arm fully extended, bend your knees to a 90 degree angle. Still keeping the kettlebell over your head, return to the starting position and repeat.

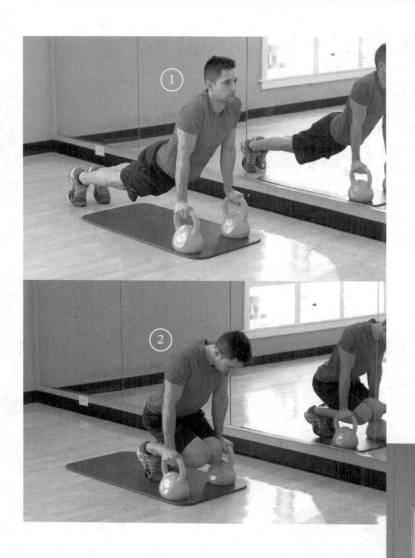

BURPEES

REPS: 10

DESCRIPTION/NOTES: Begin in the push-up position with a kettlebell in each hand. With your weight on the kettlebells, bring your knees and feet up to your chest and, in one fluid motion, spring upwards into the standing position with the kettlebells at your sides. From the standing position, squat back down and place both kettlebells on the floor, then thrust your legs out behind you back into the original push-up position.

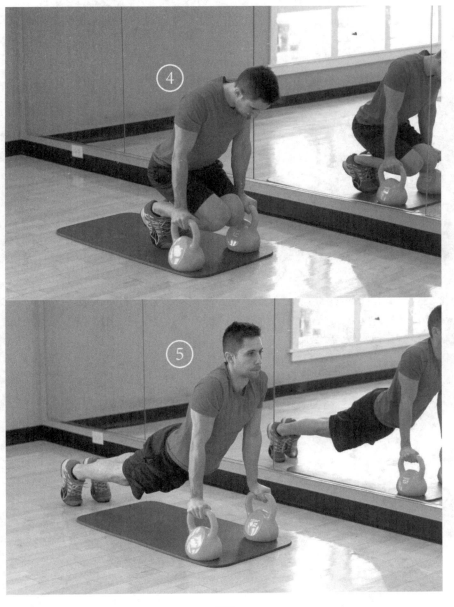

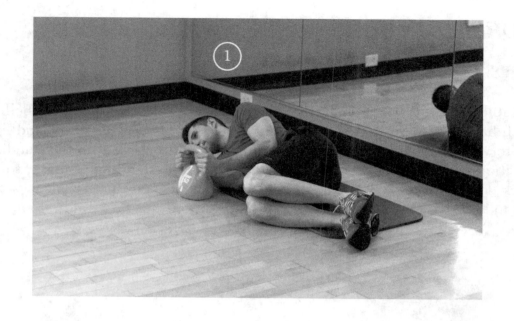

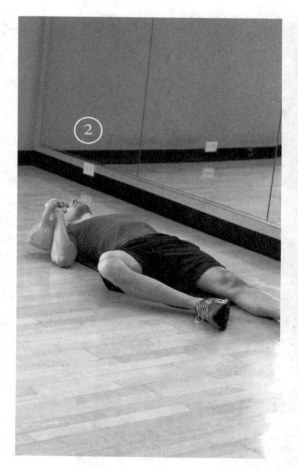

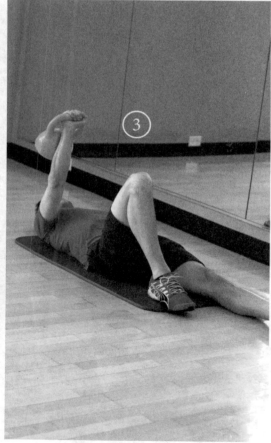

GET-UPS

REPS: 5 REPS ON EACH SIDE

DESCRIPTION/NOTES: Lie on your side in the fetal position and hold one kettlebell with both hands. Roll onto your back with the kettlebell now in one hand. Fully extend the kettlebell above your chest with one leg bent as you prepare to stand up. With the assistance of your off-hand pushing against the floor, begin to stand up with the kettlebell held above your head. Once you are standing upright with your arm full extended above your head, you will want to reverse the process to get back into the starting position to repeat.

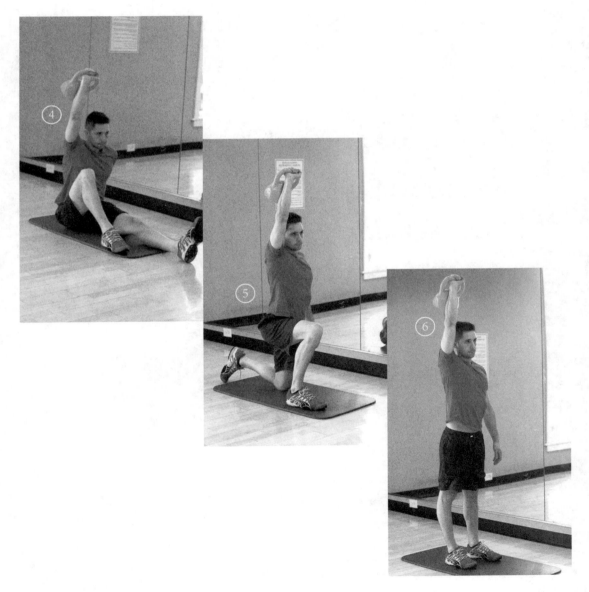

ONWARDS TO GLORY

Kettlebells are a fantastic piece of affordable gym equipment.

Used as part of a varied workout routine, they can really help to deliver the exercise goals you want to achieve.

I hope this book has shown that whether you want to get supremely fit, build muscle, or lose fat; kettlebells can really help.

The Key "Take-Aways"

- Compared to gym machines and bench exercises, kettlebells make you work harder for each rep.

- Kettlebells provide a great combination of strength, flexibility and endurance training.

- Remember; **Bad Technique = Increased Chance of Injury**. Maintain good technique and use the correct kettlebell weight that is suitable for you. This will lead to more successful results.

- Always maintain a neutral spine position. Keep your grip in a neutral position so your wrist neither flexes nor extends. Keep your center of gravity around your abdominal area. Drive through with your legs and hips when lifting the kettlebell from a low position to a high position.

- Incorporating Kettlebell exercises into your established workouts is a great way to keep your training fresh and interesting.

Happy Kettlebelling!!

THE AUTHOR

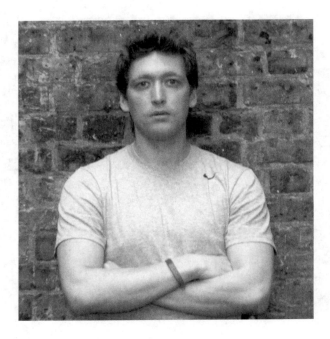

Jim McHale is an endurance athlete with experience competing in Ironman Triathlon and long distance endurance events including the 190km Libyan Challenge Desert Race.

Jim has been designing strength and cardiovascular gym circuits for well over 10 years. He has an unhealthy obsession with all areas of fitness and nutrition!

In 2010, Jim also co-authored the book *Hardcore Circuit Training for Men* which can be found in bookstores worldwide and online.

Training Notes

Training Notes

Training Notes

Training Notes

Training Notes

Training Notes

MUSCLE EXPLOSION

28 DAYS TO MAXIMUM MASS

If you are part of the "conventional wisdom crowd", take a very deep breath... with Muscle Explosion you're going to:

- Reduce caloric intake to well below maintenance levels and eliminate protein completely (in very specific ways for very specific purposes)
- Aim to overtrain
- Train the same body part five days in a row
- Perform the same exercise five days in a row

Muscle Explosion literally turns conventional muscle-building wisdom inside-out and upside down. By practicing the groundbreaking training and eating strategies in this book, you will SHATTER your ""genetic limitations"" by literally changing your physiology, quickly setting the stage for EXPLOSIVE increases in muscle mass and strength.

Each cycle of this program lasts only 28 days and the workouts take less than an hour to complete. This book is for the intermediate to advanced trainer who is ready to DEMOLISH plateaus and achieve growth and strength increases previously thought unattainable.

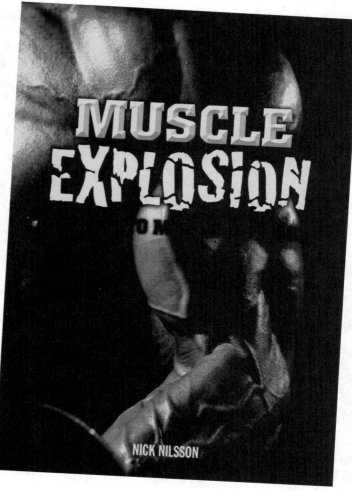

ISBN-13:	978-0-9724102-9-8
Retail Price:	$14.95
Size:	7" x 10"
Page Count:	224

About the Author

Nick Nilsson, "The Mad Scientist" of the fitness world, is a renowned personal trainer, body builder, and professional fitness writer who has written for Men's Fitness, Reps Magazine, Muscle & Fitness and hundreds of fitness websites all over the internet. He is recognized throughout the fitness world as an innovator and pioneer of ground-breaking methods for building muscle and strength fast. His degree in physical education covers advanced biomechanics, physiology and kinesiology.

SPECIAL OFFER

Get this book for 50% off (only $7.48) at **SportsWorkout.com** by using coupon code **HCME** during checkout

Pure Physique

How to MAXIMIZE Fat-Loss- and Musclular Development

Pure Physique is for anyone who ever felt they should be getting more from their efforts in and out of the gym. This book will teach you how to put together an exercise and nutrition program that is truly tailor-fitted to meet your individual needs and goals. Unlike other books that provide fad diets and 'canned' workout routines, Pure Physique was designed with the individual in mind. With this book, you will finally be able obtain the leaner, more muscular body you've always wanted.

Unlike most books in the exercise and nutrition market, this book addresses how to account for differences in needs, goals, abilities, limitations, and preferences.

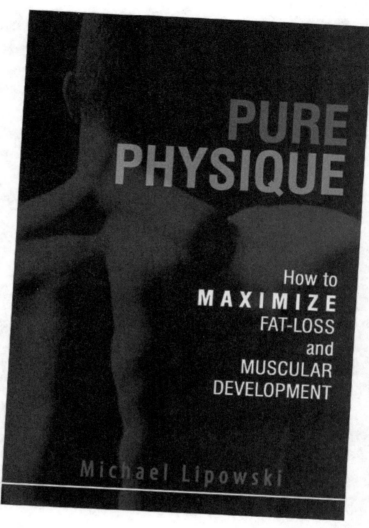

About the Author

Michael Lipowski is a certified fitness clinician and the President of the International Association of Resistance Trainers. He is a competitive natural Bodybuilder in the INBF, a consultant to other drug-free body builders, and was the personal trainer of the winner of the 2009 Men's Fitness Fit-to-Fat competition. Michael is a writer for Natural Bodybuilding & Fitness and has written for a number of other health and fitness publications worldwide.

ISBN-13:	978-0-9724102-7-4
Retail Price:	$14.95
Size:	7" x 10"
Page Count:	224

SPECIAL OFFER

Get this book for 50% off (only $7.48) at **SportsWorkout.com** by using coupon code **HCPURE** during checkout

INDEX

A

abdominal, 17, 83, 138

ability, 17, 31, 43, 57, 71, 83, 95, 107, 117, 127

act, 13

activities, 15

activity, 23

aerobic, 15, 31, 107, 117

aligned, 103

alignment, 17

alternating, 33

application, 2

areas, 15, 25, 141

arms, 33, 37, 39, 41, 47, 49, 59, 67, 75, 79, 85, 87, 89, 93, 99, 109, 119, 129

assistance, 69, 135

athlete, 141

athletes, 13

B

balanced, 37, 53, 85

barbells, 13

beginners, 17, 31, 107

beginning, 2, 29

bench, 15, 138

bending, 103, 125

bicep, 31

bikes, 13

biomechanics, 148

bolt, 71

breaking, 148

breaks, 15

breath, 148

burning, 9, 107, 117, 127

burpees, 57, 95, 117, 127

buttocks, 17

fitness, 2, 31, 43, 57, 71, 83, 95, 107, 117, 127, 141, 148

flexibility, 15, 138

fluid, 45, 63, 73, 77, 101, 105, 121, 123, 133

G

gravity, 17, 138

gym, 5, 13, 15, 137-138, 141

H

handle, 13, 17

hands, 37, 39, 47, 49, 65, 69, 73, 75, 79, 85, 87, 89, 91, 109, 119, 129, 135

hazardous, 17

height, 35, 75

hips, 17, 105, 138

holding, 33, 35, 41, 53, 55, 59, 73, 75, 77, 79, 97, 103, 115, 131

I

ideal, 23, 27, 31, 57, 107, 127

improving, 17

injury, 2, 17, 21

innovator, 148

instructions, 31, 43, 83, 95, 107, 117, 127

intake, 148

intensity, 15, 23, 27

intermediate, 148

interval, 15, 57

J

jogging, 23

joint, 17

K

kettlebelling, 138

kinesiology, 148

knees, 37, 45, 47, 55, 63, 65, 67, 85, 91, 93, 97, 101, 105, 109, 113, 115, 119, 121, 123, 125, 129, 131, 133

L

lactic, 27

legs, 17, 37, 39, 41, 45, 47, 49, 51, 63, 65, 67, 77, 85, 87, 89, 91, 93, 99, 101, 109, 113, 119, 121, 123, 125, 129, 133, 138

lower, 59, 61, 81, 111

lunges, 43, 95